I0420283

Where Can I Find Miscarriage Support?

Personal Story By:

Kris Cottrell

The information found in and through MiscarriageSupport.com is for general purposes only. Information found through this eBook and through the MiscarriageSupport.com Website should NOT be construed as definitive or binding advice. MiscarriageSupport.com is not a professional therapy service. We simply provide our story and ways that we found help through a difficult time.

Reproduction of any material contained in MiscarriageSupport.com is prohibited.

MiscarriageSupport.com is under NO obligation and does not assume any obligation to monitor the information residing on or transmitted to this service.

Disclaimer of Liability:

THE USE OF ANY RECOMMENDED SERVICE PROVIDERS ASSUMES ALL RESPONSIBILITY AND RISK FOR THE USE OF THIS SERVICE AND THE INTERNET GENERALLY. MISCARRIAGESUPPORT.COM DISCLAIMS ALL WARRANTIES, EXPRESS OR IMPLIED, WITH REGARD TO THE INFORMATION ACCESSED FROM, OR VIA, THIS SERVICE OR INTERNET, INCLUDING, BUT NOT LIMITED TO, ALL IMPLIED WARRANTIES OF MERCHANTABILITY, OR NON-INFRINGEMENT.

THE MISCARRIAGESUPPORT.COM DOES NOT ASSUME ANY LEGAL LIABILITY OR RESPONSIBILITY FOR THE ACCURACY, COMPLETENESS, OR USEFULNESS OF ANY INFORMATION, APPARATUS, PRODUCT OR PROCESS DISCLOSED ON THE SERVICE OR OTHER MATERIAL ACCESSIBLE FROM THE SERVICE. IN NO EVENT SHALL THE MISCARRIAGESUPPORT.COM BE LIABLE FOR ANY SPECIAL, INDIRECT, OR CONSEQUENTIAL DAMAGES OR ANY DAMAGES WHATSOEVER RESULTING FROM LOSS OF USE, DATA, OR PROFITS, WHETHER IN AN ACTION OF CONTRACT, NEGLIGENCE OR OTHERWISE, ARISING OUT OF OR IN CONNECTION WITH THE USE OR PERFORMANCE OF THE INFORMATION ON THIS SERVICE OR THE INTERNET GENERALLY.

Any material contained on this service may include inaccuracies or errors.

THE INFORMATION PROVIDED ON THIS SERVICE IS PROVIDED ON AN "AS IS" AND "AS AVAILABLE" BASIS WITHOUT WARRANTIES OF ANY KIND, EITHER EXPRESSED OR IMPLIED, INCLUDING BUT NOT LIMITED TO WARRANTIES OF TITLE, NON-INFRINGEMENT OR IMPLIED WARRANTIES OF MERCHANTABILITY FOR A PARTICULAR PURPOSE. ALL USERS OF THIS SERVICE AGREE TO HOLD HARMLESS THE MISCARRIAGESUPPORT.COM, ITS PRINCIPLES AND OWNERS, FROM ANY CLAIMS WHATSOEVER, INCLUDING LOSSES, EXPENSES, AND REASONABLE ATTORNEY FEES ARISING FROM THE USE OF THIS SERVICE. NO ADVICE OR INFORMATION GIVEN BY THE MISCARRIAGESUPPORT.COM SHALL CREATE ANY WARRANTY.

Why Did I Write This eBook?

I n March of 2001, after a five month pregnancy and with great anticipation of another child, my wife and I experienced a miscarriage. We were devastated. My wife Robin was especially heartbroken. She had bonded with this unborn child through months of sickness, feeling the baby move within her and hours of eager preparation in our home for a newborn. There was no warning and no inner promptings of any kind. Everything appeared on schedule medically, emotionally and spiritually. We had no idea how deeply our lives would be forever changed.

My desire in writing this book is to share our experience, our knowledge and our understanding that helped us heal from our miscarriage. Miscarriages come suddenly with very little insight and minimal empathy or sympathy from anyone or anywhere. Our goal is to provide hope to couples experiencing these tragic losses of unborn children.

For months after the miscarriage, my wife spent hours online and in bookstores searching for answers and help but found very little. Some websites had products to buy or stories of others who also experienced miscarriages, but none of them provided quite the understanding that we received through prayer and pondering for years since our miscarriage. Outside of potential medical reasons for the miscarriage, there was no information and nowhere, other than our faith and our love for each other, to find help to heal.

We've learned many things through this experience. The first is that you don't have to do this alone. You will feel like you're in a very lonely place, yet being alone will only compound the pain. **There are <u>over 600,000</u> miscarriages reported each year in the United States, and many more are not reported**. Not only are many not reported they are also typically not even spoken of outside the home. There seems to be almost a feeling of shame talking about a miscarriage. I learned there is literally an army of men and women walking around us each day who have felt the crushing blow of a miscarriage. They too have had their dreams shattered and now possess a daily fear of trying again to have a child. They understand that aching in the heart that just doesn't go away. They also feel the pain when seeing other pregnant women or young couples holding their newborns.

Though many share this experience, very few talk about it openly. It is difficult to talk about something that wasn't "real" to others. Unless you have experienced a miscarriage you really cannot understand. In addition, most people don't know how to react or what to say; and that makes sharing something so personal even more uncomfortable. It's ironic that one of the very things that helps us heal from a miscarriage IS talking about it, particularly communication between husband and wife, boyfriend and girlfriend.

Robin and I are not ashamed or uncomfortable talking about it! **Our goal is to help you and others like you begin a healing process that may take years.** The following pages contain principles we have learned that we pray will bring you hope and strength.

To your happiness and healing,

Kris Cottrell

Online Videos, Articles, Modules, Stories, Forum, Webinars, Question and Answers and Interviews

To help you heal…

http://www.MiscarriageSupport.com

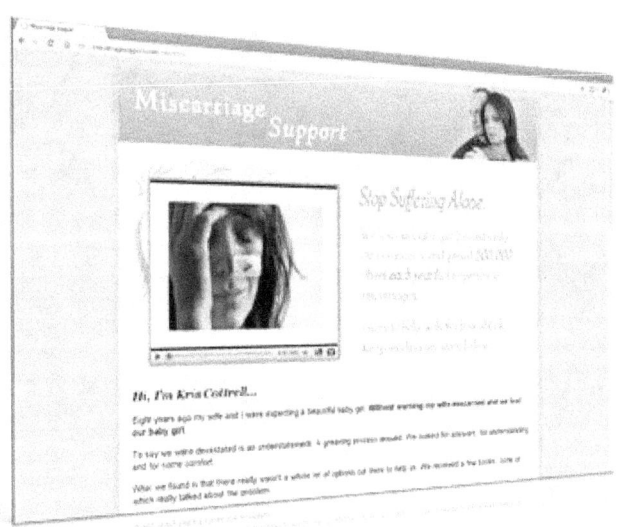

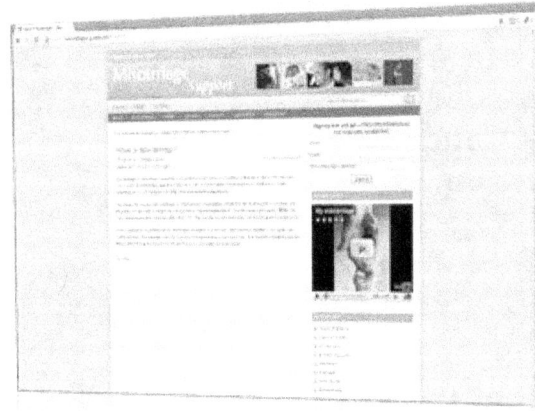

We know how difficult this time can be.

To listen to a message of hope and healing join us at

MiscarriageSupport.com

To obtain access to our membership site, please email:

support@miscarriagesupport.com

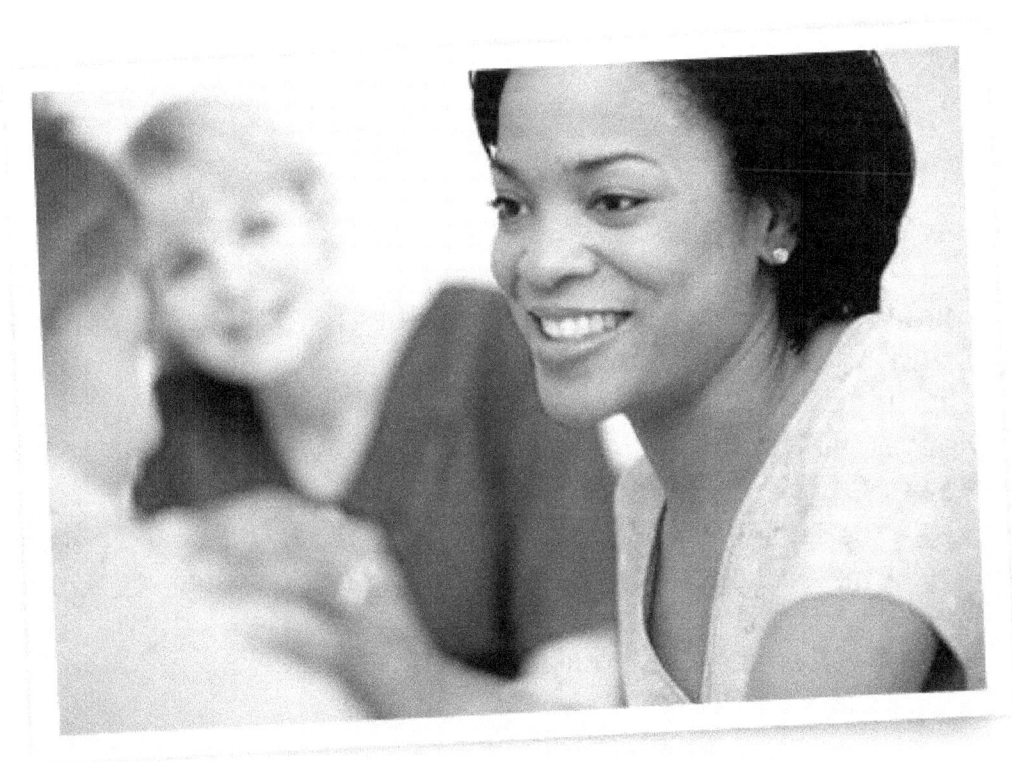

Table of Contents

Copyright © 2009 MiscarriageSupport.com

Get Professional Support... call 1-800-275-9105

Copyright © 2009 **MiscarriageSupport.com**

Get Professional Support... call 1-800-275-9105

Chapter One

Many years ago I attended a scout camp in the deep wilderness of Wyoming. As a thirteen year old I came up with an entertaining game called log tag. The rules of log tag are simple: Each scout has to stay on top of the wet, fallen logs and play tag. If you fall off or if you're tagged, you're it. I fully believed I was the most athletic scout and could easily win this game. What I hadn't taken into consideration was that the logs were very slippery when wet and that it rains nearly every day in the Rocky Mountains. During one game I was running from log to log to get away, and as I went to jump to a distant log I slipped and fell. My right leg landed on a small pine tree another scout had widdled into a standing spear. The sharp, pointy tree went into my leg just below the knee. I was stuck! I had to pull my leg off of the tree to free myself. I was in shock!

This cool game that I had invented and was excited about just resulted in me pulling my leg off of a tree imbedded halfway through my calf. Once I got my leg off the tree I was overcome with deep throbbing pain. It really, really hurt. I tried to be tough. However, fear, pain and shock caused me to shed a few tears. This left a very deep, wide hole in my leg. It was bleeding badly and I began to feel queasy. I reluctantly went for some help, as I knew I couldn't fix this injury by myself. Upon seeing my injury my scout leaders drove me on a dirt road to the nearest town which was forty miles away.

We arrived in Afton, Wyoming, where I was taken into the emergency room and introduced to someone who could help me. A kind doctor put his arm around me and told me it would be okay. He seemed to really understand the situation I was in and the frightening feelings I was experiencing. The first thing he did was to

Copyright © 2009 **MiscarriageSupport.com**

Get Professional Support... call 1-800-275-9105

begin washing it out with a sterile solution and cleaning the wound. This really hurt! He put in some fluid that really stung. It actually felt almost as bad as the pain of pulling my leg off the little tree. Once it was cleaned, scrubbed and had antibiotics dumped into it, he sewed up my leg with a needle and thread. He put a bandage on it and sent me on my way.

I felt so much better after leaving the hospital. However, the wound hurt for a long time and it took a year to heal. The pain didn't completely leave after I left the hospital. It would often throb at night and hurt when it got bumped. Finally, the stitches were removed and a scab formed. Sometimes during everyday life the scab would be torn off, and the wound would bleed again. Finally, the wound began to completely heal but left one very tender spot on my leg. It eventually turned into a beautiful scar that I still sport today! The area around the scar is still numb.

The great news is that I can still use that leg. It works just fine like it did before. I do have a reminder that the enjoyment of log tag can also be hurtful. This reminder now helps me teach my kids and others to be careful about playing log tag. It hasn't stopped me from inventing new fun and interesting games or laughing at myself. I enjoy life as much as I did before the accident.

I learned that my entire healing process was controlled by a higher power. I went through the steps that I knew of to help my leg heal, but I was not the healer. After many years I'm doing very well regardless of this traumatic experience when I was thirteen.

As I look back on this experience and ponder it, I realize that there is a process that our bodies go through when they are injured. First we go into shock. Then we experience pain, blood, tears and the need to get assistance from others. The wound must be cleaned and sterilized, sewn up, scabbed over and, eventually, marked with a scar.

The body and the spirit are the soul of man. Therefore, the healing process that our spirit goes through when it hurts is very similar to the healing process of our physical bodies. We heal emotionally exactly the same way we heal physically.

Copyright © 2009 **MiscarriageSupport.com**
Get Professional Support... call 1-800-275-9105

Each chapter in this book will discuss the healing process as it relates to the wound your soul encountered experiencing a miscarriage.

Copyright © 2009 **MiscarriageSupport.com**

Get Professional Support... call 1-800-275-9105

Chapter

Shock And Disappointment

As careful as a pregnant women is with her health, there is always a chance of her experiencing a miscarriage. Current statistics show that one in four pregnancies ends in a miscarriage. Some think that number is closer to one in three. So statistically, if you are going to have a family, odds are that you may experience one or more miscarriages.

When a miscarriage occurs, the mother AND the father are overwhelmed with grief and pain. It is devastating. Not only is there shock that the baby has died and you don't know what to do; but there is also surprise at what options there are to physically take care of the miscarried child. All choices for removing the baby are undesirable choices. Either the mother can give birth to the deceased fetus, or the doctor can perform a D&C and take the fetus from the mother via surgery. These are both tough options, especially after just receiving the news about the baby. Make sure you listen to your doctor; and if you haven't consulted one, make sure you do. They have a lot of experience with miscarriages and will give you the best options available. It can be very dangerous not to consult a physician during or after a miscarriage. I believe they will be very sensitive to your situation and provide guidance to help you.

Just as I realized I had to tell someone about my wound from playing log tag, the thoughts of now having to tell a lot of people about a miscarriage can compound the experience. This can feel overwhelming. The last thing that you feel like doing is calling family and friends and discussing the circumstances of the miscarriage. Many of them may not have even known you were pregnant.

Copyright © 2009 **MiscarriageSupport.com**

Get Professional Support... call 1-800-275-9105

It is important to remember all of these feelings are completely normal. Nobody likes or wants to answer questions about their personal lives, especially around something so emotional. I learned it is okay to feel this way. If you don't feel like talking about it immediately afterwards, then don't! Listen to your feelings. Your heart will tell you what to do. You have been born with an inner compass that will guide you throughout your life if you will learn to trust it. It is okay to begin grieving and dealing with your loss the way YOU want. Remember, you have the same amount of control healing your inside as you do your outside. You can and should make choices based on your thoughts and feelings.

There are things you can do to help to keep this emotional wound from getting "infected." Remember, even though you do all you can to heal, you are not the healer. Your spirit will take over and heal the wound from the inside out. In other words this emotional wound will be healed AFTER all you can do. Do all you can and then know your natural inside or spirit will do the rest! Have hope and know you will make it through this. You don't typically worry about your physical wounds healing over. They just gradually do. You also don't need to worry about your emotional wounds healing over, if and only if you properly care for the wound. If you have no one to lean on, please call LeanOnUs 1-877-532-6668. This number rings into counselors who can help you for a very economical price.

Copyright © 2009 **MiscarriageSupport.com**

Get Professional Support... call 1-800-275-9105

Deep And Incredible Pain

Pain and sadness come when we lose a child. There is no way around it. It is a natural byproduct of love. When we lose someone we love, our heart, mind and soul hurt. This is really our spirit within us being pained. Just like a physical wound these inner spiritual and emotional wounds hurt the most at the time the wound occurs. Over time the pain will dissipate. It never leaves altogether, but it will not be as sharp as it was in the beginning. The love and longing for your child will never fade. Society seems to teach that those who suffer a miscarriage can be dismissed as not needing to mourn at all. This is not true. You will need to mourn the loss in your own way and time frame.

Unless a person has experienced a miscarriage firsthand she really doesn't understand. My wife had many good people come to our door and say things like, "Well at least you can try again," or "At least you're blessed to have four healthy children!" or "Something was obviously wrong with the child or this wouldn't have happened." Some even went so far as to make her feel as if she should just "get over it" and move forward. You will find that unless someone has experienced a miscarriage herself it is impossible for her to truly understand. Therefore, many may not be in a position to validate your feelings. Remember, people can only give what they have. If there truly is no understanding or experience on their part, how can you expect them to know how to comfort you in this situation? It is impossible for them. You will need to lower your expectation of what others can give you. People are doing the best they can with what they know. The fact that they are trying to comfort, trying to "be there" for you, should speak for itself, even if they do a less than a satisfactory job at it.

Each of the visitors to our home was a very good person. However, true empathy only comes with understanding. One can only truly have empathy for another if

Copyright © 2009 **MiscarriageSupport.com**

Get Professional Support... call 1-800-275-9105

and when one understands. Those who had experienced a miscarriage were much more empathic than those who hadn't. And those who spent the time to just listen and try to understand were more empathic than those who wouldn't be patient, listen and try to validate.

I've learned that the following formula is true:

Understanding → Empathy → Charity/Forgiveness

Increased understanding brings increased empathy, and increased empathy brings increased forgiveness. For those of you who may be Christians, this is why Christ had to descend below all things. It is why He had to feel everyone's pains, sicknesses, anxieties, troubles, temptations, sadnesses, etc. Otherwise, He would not have perfect empathy to help us with our situations. He is the only one who truly understands what we are going through, because He personally went through the same thing! Therefore, because He has perfect empathy for our situations, He can quickly forgive us, because He understands perfectly why we made the choices we've made. He is the one person who realizes that we are all really "good" inside. Within each of us is Godly DNA, and He can see it.

Husbands, you have a very significant role in helping your wife heal. Next to God you should be the best listener and validator to whom your wife has access. A good lesson for husbands to learn is when your wife is upset or hurting, just take the time to simply listen to her. Try to understand her. Listen with your eyes for feeling, and reflect it. Your wife isn't looking for you to fix the problem. She typically only wants you to understand her. You can help her the most through this difficult time by being sensitive to her needs. Her first and foremost need in this situation is you understanding her feelings.

Copyright © 2009 **MiscarriageSupport.com**

Get Professional Support... call 1-800-275-9105

Chapter 4

Tears Are A Natural Process For Healthy Healing.

We weep for those we lose because we love them. If there were no tears there would be no love. The fact is that you love your unborn child. You have bonded with this child within you. This child is literally a part of you, and I believe he or she always has been. You have a desire to cry as a way to express feelings of love for this child.

Tears are a way of cleansing yourself emotionally. Studies show that tears actually contain healing chemicals that help the brain. When tears are released, so are emotional toxins. Have you ever just felt like you needed a good cry, and afterward you felt much better? I do that all the time. I find myself feeling bad or hurting inside from something dumb I've done or someone else has done to me; I may try to hold it in; but eventually it just bubbles out. I typically cry while I'm driving; and yes, the cars passing by my truck wonder what in the world is wrong with this guy! But I find it feels better when I let the tears flow.

After a miscarriage you may not be able to control the flow of tears. It is okay to cry, and it is okay to cry everyday or once in a while or for many years to come. We are all different. Just remember tears are a big part of the healing process. Picture your tears as washing away the pain.

Tears are comprised of water and salt. They come from the windows of the soul-the eyes. Water is used to clean things. For instance, we shower or bathe in water to get clean. We use a hose with water to clean our cars, driveways, etc. Tears

Copyright © 2009 **MiscarriageSupport.com**

Get Professional Support... call 1-800-275-9105

clean emotional wounds just as the doctor cleaned out my leg many years ago, your spirit will clean out this deep wound with water. The spiritual doctor rinsing out the wounded soul always overflows water from the eyes.

Water is also a sign of life. Things only grow where there is water; things don't grow without it. Trees, shrubs and grasses grow along the rivers. We all need water to live, to grow and to be healthy. Suffering is an essential part of growth. It is one reason we are here. Only through suffering can we become better, stronger and more useful to others. When there are tears, there is growth. Tears come at a cost; and yet, they are essential to learn the lessons of life that perfect us. After suffering through a miscarriage, you can now lift and build others where before you had no empathy or influence to do so. You will now possess a new form of charity for others.

The tears that drop to the ground after a miscarriage are sacred. These tears come through sacrifice and pain, and you will be rewarded with a power and influence you otherwise would not have. Salt adds flavor to things. You are also becoming more valuable or flavorful to others. You will find yourself in situations over the years to help others or your own children through similar losses. You cannot lift others to higher ground unless you are already on higher ground yourself!

Nobody wants to hear that suffering is a good thing. I understand that. Yet, I see no other way for us to become a diamond from a piece of coal without the heat and pressures of the day. A great man once said that his life was like a boulder rolling down a hill. As it crashed into other rocks a sharp edge was taken off- and against a tree, another one was made smooth- until at the bottom of the hill, he became a smooth and polished stone to be used in the hand of the Master. Isn't that exactly how you feel? Life was rolling along just great; and then, "bang," you crashed into a boulder; then, "wham," you slammed into a tree. A bit of pride is knocked off here, a little bit of unthankfulness is scratched away there. Your tears are a sign of this refinement. As difficult and painful as these things are that you're slamming into, when you slow down or stop rolling through this trial, you will find yourself much more polished and refined and, therefore, much more useful to others.

Copyright © 2009 **MiscarriageSupport.com**

Get Professional Support... call 1-800-275-9105

Chapter 5

Blaming Myself

I thought to myself, upon finding my leg stuck to a tree at age thirteen, "I am such an idiot. Why do I always do dumb things? Why did this have to happen to me? I never should have thought up this dumb game and forced everyone to play it. I've ruined everyone else's camp, because now I can't join in the other activities." And so on. I was blaming myself for this pain I was in.

You may be having thoughts like: "I shouldn't have walked around all day the day before my miscarriage. I should have stayed away from those cleaning chemicals. I knew I was overdoing it with that activity. I shouldn't have put myself in that stressful situation. I feel extreme guilt because of my own actions. I feel I may have contributed in some way to this awful experience."

These are normal feelings of shame and blaming yourself. The truth is there is typically no way to tell the exact cause of the miscarriage. You cannot truthfully blame yourself for causing a miscarriage; because, most likely, you will never fully know why. You didn't cause the miscarriage. A much higher power was involved in the decision. Sorry, but you aren't that capable. If you were, you could have stopped this from happening. Think about it!

Rather than try and find or place blame, look forward with faith.

Remember, "It isn't the snakebite that killed the man; it was chasing the snake around afterward to chop its head off that drove the poison to the heart." This includes your own heart. You will do far more damage trying to attach blame somewhere than moving forward and learning from the experience. Rather than blame yourself, why not think, "What am I suppose to learn from this experience?" "How can I become better because of this?" As I've mentioned,

Copyright © 2009 **MiscarriageSupport.com**

Get Professional Support... call 1-800-275-9105

understanding brings empathy, and empathy brings forgiveness, even when we think we need to forgive ourselves.

I believe that if you will ponder and pray about what has happened to you, you will gradually gain some insight that you currently don't possess. I don't believe this miscarriage has happened to you because you did something wrong. I believe things happen to give us experience and to help us grow in ways we couldn't without these experiences.

Copyright © 2009 **MiscarriageSupport.com**

Get Professional Support... call 1-800-275-9105

Oftentimes We Need Other's Help To Make Us Feel Better.

I needed to find help when I hurt my leg. I couldn't have limped forty miles to a doctor on a mountainous dirt road. Most of the time you will also need help to heal. It is very important to be able to talk to someone. I recommend you talk to your spouse. You are in a relationship for a reason. Often the husband doesn't take as long to recover from a miscarriage and can sometimes be curt or impatient as the woman processes through the experience. If you will be patient with each other and go through the loss and healing process together, it will deepen and improve your relationship.

Husbands need to realize a miscarriage isn't something that women just "get over." You cannot go around or under the feelings of a miscarriage. You have to go through them. Eventually, you will feel all of this emotional pain and find on the other side a peace and healing that will improve and purify you, if you let it.

Robin was at a drive-up, fast-food window weeks after her miscarriage. The young man at the window was taking her money, when she heard herself blurt out, "I just had a miscarriage!" The young man looked at her bewildered and shut the window. Robin was embarrassed and wondered why she said that to a complete stranger. This simply shows the need to get these feelings out to someone. You will need others to help.

Copyright © 2009 **MiscarriageSupport.com**

Get Professional Support... call 1-800-275-9105

Chapter

7

Cleaning The Wound

When I went to the doctor for my leg, the first thing he did was to clean the wound. He used water and antibiotics. Each of our wounds must be cleaned out. Without a cleansing process, infection will result. Infection could lead to larger problems or even death.

Emotional and spiritual wounds require the same cleansing process as physical wounds. This is accomplished by talking about what happened. Just as a doctor cleans and disinfects a physical wound, you also cleanse an emotional wound by talking openly about it. Just as my leg hurt terribly when the doctor was scrubbing it and administering antibiotics to kill any possible infection, so talking about something so sacred and painful can be excruciating. You need to talk to those who support and love you. Talk to your spouse, a parent, a pastor or a close friend.

Talk about your experience, your pain, your feelings and your thoughts. Talking brings clarity to your mind. It will help bring closure, even though you may think just the opposite. You may feel that speaking about what happened will keep it in front of you; there is actually a therapeutic result in processing or thinking out loud about your situation when you feel the need. Your story is real to you; it isn't real to others. When you don't get the response back you hoped for, you need to remember this: You experienced this, they didn't. It is your child you lost, not theirs.

You will have the temptation to isolate and be alone. It is a natural feeling to want to just hide in your bed when tough times come. This is okay in small doses. But resist the continual feeling to isolate. Long-term isolation will not help you heal.

13

Copyright © 2009 **MiscarriageSupport.com**

Get Professional Support... call 1-800-275-9105

You need to be engaged with others to the extent you can stand it. Brief periods of isolation may be healthy, but prolonged isolation causes infection.

My wife had a dream regarding a painful situation in her life. In the dream she had a cast on her leg. The cast was unraveling; and, thus, the hurt part of her leg was exposed and not able to completely heal. Days later she shared this wonderful insight with me. She felt like the cast was being unwoven because it was so dry. It needed to be moistened with water. It needed "living water" that only comes from God by listening to your thoughts and impressions. You must keep the cast wet; or it will dry out and unravel, exposing your painful parts. The following are some ways to keep water on your emotional cast. They are ideas that will help keep moist bandages on your gaping, emotional, miscarriage wound.

Journaling

Journaling is one of the most therapeutic activities you can do to heal from any emotional wound. A journal can become a best friend who always understands, never has anything bad to say to you and always wants to absorb your feelings. Journal as often as you feel a need to express yourself. Journaling is a personal and safe way to get your feelings out. It is a way to express your thoughts and feelings on paper. Writing forces clarity. When something in your mind is not clear, then write about it. The thought or idea will become clearer as it is written. I am much more effective teaching or brainstorming when I have a whiteboard and marker; because I learn through clarification: and the concepts grow as I write them. I can see the thoughts and principles on the board. They begin to take shape, to become almost alive in my mind and on the board. I can then more easily build upon those thoughts. We recommend you write and write consistently. When you need to let out feelings and there isn't anyone to visit with, tell your journal.

Video Journal

A simple flip camera for around one hundred dollars is a great way to make a video journal or blog. Simply put the camera in front of you, and turn it on. Give updates on how you feel, and over time you can watch your old videos and recognize the improvement to your mental and emotional health. Then simply

Copyright © 2009 **MiscarriageSupport.com**

Get Professional Support... call 1-800-275-9105

plug it into your computer, and it is uploaded in minutes to burn on a DVD or place on a storage device. This is also a great way to help your posterity with challenges. We have an opportunity to teach others from our experiences. Video journaling is a way to capture feeling along with your story. It is you talking about your personal struggles and triumphs. Someday, I guarantee someone will be going through a similar challenge and will be lifted and will gain hope from your experience, if it is documented and if you desire to share it.

Scrapbooking

Scrapbooking is another proactive activity available to help you. Start with your ultrasound, if you were far enough along to have an ultrasound, and if the doctor printed the picture of your baby. If not, you may want to scrapbook your feelings. Make a collage of your pregnancy, your marriage and your relationship with your spouse. Scrapbooking a baby page can also be moisture to your emotional cast.

Music

Soft, uplifting music can heal the soul. The opposite is true with non-uplifting music. It will bring anxiousness, depression and sad feelings. Classical music helps the frontal lobe and will make you feel more peaceful. Play soft uplifting music in your home continually. Play it in your car, while you walk or while you eat dinner.

Examples of therapeutic music we find healing include: classical music, instrumental music (such as Yanni or Jim Brickman) and fun uplifting music like (James Taylor). Play music that YOU find soothing to YOUR soul. This can be different things to different people. I would recommend you stay away from hard rock or rap music that may bring anxiety or nervous tension to you. As you know, music carries certain beats and rhythms. Beats and rhythms make us feel things. Our nervous system and our mind react to the beats and rhythms of music. Some are uplifting, calming and relaxing. Others bring tension, anxiousness and even aggressiveness. Remember, there is great power in the music you have around you. If you're not used to listening to my recommendations, then just try them for a few weeks and see if you notice a difference. I believe you will, and it will be significant. Play it softly in the background of your day.

Copyright © 2009 **MiscarriageSupport.com**

Get Professional Support... call 1-800-275-9105

Pictures

Buy and put things around home to help you heal by visual stimulation. We put pictures of temples, Christ and other paintings to remind us of our faith and our child. Having visual pictures around the house can help lift your spirits. Often we use visual reminders to help us reach goals or inspire us. I can't think of anything more rewarding than to have reminders about eternal families, faith and our children.

Necklace: Something Tangible

My wife bought a necklace and attached a pinky ring to the necklace. This became a physical reminder to her of our child. I would often see her touching it or playing with it while it was around her neck. Many times she wasn't even aware she was doing it. It told me that she was having those feelings inside. You may choose to get one with the child's birthstone. This is very healing because you have something tangible to touch when you are thinking of your baby. This, by no means, is a replacement for the unborn child; but it is something physical you can carry with you and will help.

Name your baby.

You may choose to give your child a name. This can be a very good thing. Rather than call the child "our baby" or "our child." This real person can have a real name. This is completely up to you. Many people don't name their child. We chose not to; but naming your baby may be a healing step.

Stay busy.

Discover a new hobby, take a class and learn something new. Volunteering and helping someone else can keep you from slipping into inactivity and depression. Staying busy will also keep your mind off your grief. Find those things that are

Copyright © 2009 **MiscarriageSupport.com**
Get Professional Support... call 1-800-275-9105

uplifting to you or that help others. You will find yourself much happier when you are busy serving others or completing something you love.

Help someone else.

Simply listening to someone else can be extremely helpful to them. You are finding this out yourself. Serving others helps you forget your own problems. I've found nothing more therapeutic when we feel down, angry, depressed or anxious than serving and helping someone else with a problem. This principle is like the miracle of the loaves and the fishes. You give out a little bit of what you have in your basket to feed others, and it will return with increase. You cannot help another without helping yourself in the process. True happiness and healing cannot become yours until and unless you are willing to share it. It is by giving happiness and healing away that it becomes yours. There is great power in this principle. Look for opportunities in your home, church, school and community. Look for a cause that will motivate you. I've learned that money, competition, power or popularity are not the most powerful motivators. Having a cause for something you believe in is the one long-lasting motivator. Blessing the lives of those in need is an innate motivator that lies within our DNA. This always brings us a sense of joy. If you want to heal, first be the healer. This is why we started our website www.miscarriagesupport.com forming a miscarriage community.

One cause you may want to join is helping those who also suffer from a miscarriage. You can join us in helping others by purchasing our miscarriage recovery membership. A percentage of your contribution will go to help other families dealing with a miscarriage. Some ways your money will help them include: medical bills, comfort necklaces, birthday letters, and counseling. We are also helping to support a high-risk pregnancy clinic needing funding to be built.

Time

It's said that Time is "that great healer." The challenge is that it takes so darn long! ☺ Pain from a miscarriage won't completely leave, but it also won't be as constant over time. Pain seems to lesson with time. It is interesting to me to think that you are sad because you will not be able to spend any time with this child; and, yet, time passing will help the pain.

Copyright © 2009 **MiscarriageSupport.com**
Get Professional Support... call 1-800-275-9105

Try and remove time from your equation. I find that because of time we often beat ourselves up. For instance, I've counseled many people who feel they have failed as a parent. They may have a teenager making poor choices. I often change their paradigm when I ask them if they would still be a failed parent if their child got on the right path when he turned twenty five. They say, "Well no, I wouldn't be a failure then." I ask them if they would still be a failure if their child turned his life around when he turned sixty five. They respond the same. I then ask them, what if your child didn't turn his life around until one thousand years from now on the other side. Would you still be a failure? I answer for them, "NO. You are not a failure." Do the best you can; be always teaching; love unconditionally; and you cannot fail.

Thus, remove time from your healing equation. You will gradually heal. It may take a while, but you will eventually feel much better I promise!

Copyright © 2009 **MiscarriageSupport.com**

Get Professional Support... call 1-800-275-9105

One Day At A Time

Y ou have heard the answer to the question of how to eat an elephant- one bite at a time. When you experience a challenge in your life and you find yourself in the middle of it, break down these difficult times into shorter periods. Don't eat it all at once. Look at your day as a bunch of mini-days called hours. Get through the next hour, then the next. As you do this, you will soon put a string of days together- then weeks, then months will pass.

Planning something to look forward to will also help pass time. You were planning and looking forward to a baby with great anticipation. Find something else to plan and do, such as, a vacation, a gift you've always wanted or a remodel of a room in your house. Set a goal and work towards this. You may possibly choose to run a marathon, to grow a garden or even to advocate a cause that is meaningful to you. It will help you focus your attention on something other than the baby. It will help time move more swiftly. We like to plan our vacations well in advance and let our family know about them early. We have found that the anticipation is nearly as much fun as the vacation or family gift.

Keeping memory alive

Many people have asked about the appropriateness of naming a miscarried child. The answer is that it is entirely up to you. I believe a name can provide substance and meaning to someone not physically here. Counsel with your spouse and decide the appropriate direction for you.

Another personal decision is whether or not to have a burial spot. Once again this is a personal decision. You can contact your local mortuary, and they can provide

Copyright © 2009 **MiscarriageSupport.com**

Get Professional Support... call 1-800-275-9105

you with options. Having a final resting place can provide a lifelong place to visit and remember your little one.

Copyright © 2009 **MiscarriageSupport.com**

Get Professional Support... call 1-800-275-9105

Love What You Have And Be Grateful.

Gratitude is the magic, forgetting potient that helps us forget our troubles. I read a quote once that said, "I felt bad because I have no shoes until I saw a man with no feet!" We can be grateful for simple little things. Gratitude brings much different feelings to us than anger, sadness or depression. Concentrate and focus on what you DO have. Count your many blessings day by day and see how much you DO have. Gratitude helps to remove doubt and increases self esteem. It helps lift discouragement and parts the clouds of self-condemnation.

Be grateful you have a spouse who is trying to understand and help. No, he isn't perfect at it and often doesn't understand; but at least there is someone there trying to support you.

Be grateful for your family. No family is perfect, but it is the most important thing we have. When we die we only take with us two things: our experiences and our relationships we've formed. Live each day remembering that relationships are the most important thing you have, and it will change the way you treat people. Relationships are much more important than work, money or things. Treat your family as the best gift you will ever have; because it is. Be thankful for your family. This will help you heal.

Keep a gratitude journal. By writing down each day those things that went well or God's hand in your life, you will begin to see a pattern of tender mercies that continually happen to you daily. This will keep you from focusing on the negative things in your life. You will find you begin to talk and think more positive

Copyright © 2009 **MiscarriageSupport.com**

Get Professional Support... call 1-800-275-9105

thoughts as you focus on the good and not the bad. By writing them down, you will easily see patterns and have a great reference book to look back on during dark emotional days.

Copyright © 2009 **MiscarriageSupport.com**

Get Professional Support... call 1-800-275-9105

Chapter

10

Scab: An Outward Sign of Healing

It always takes much longer than we want it to. Just as my leg began to heal, so will your heart. Gradually, the wound begins to not hurt as badly. It begins to feel better and better ever so gradually.

Scabs form when wounds are healing. Scabs are hard shells formed over a wound. They form a protective helmet, making the wound less sensitive and keeping the wound from bleeding and from further infection. Your emotional and spiritual wound will also form a scab, not one you can see but others may see it. You will not be as sensitive as you were at first. You may not cry quite as often. You won't feel as if your heart is completely open and bleeding as you do now. There will form a protective coating, helping you to be less sensitive to bumping this wound. Bumps happen when you see babies, when people make comments or when you see something that reminds you of your baby. Sometimes, just like my leg your emotional scab will get bumped and start to bleed again. This may result in painful feelings, crying and depression. Remember, the torn scab heals much faster than the gaping, open wound. It still hurts badly: but it closes up much, much faster. Scabs are another tender mercy to help us heal.

Copyright © 2009 **MiscarriageSupport.com**

Get Professional Support... call 1-800-275-9105

Scarring

The last stage of the healing process is scarring. I still carry the scar on my leg from when I was thirteen as a reminder of my experience. You, too, will always carry a scar on your heart and on your soul. It will serve as a reminder and a protection. It is a battle wound of life. It represents a very difficult time in your life that you *made it through*. It holds within it wisdom and knowledge that can come only through pain and sacrifice. It can be used to bless and help others going through similar times. You bear the mark or token now as one who understands. There is no greater power or influence than that. Move forward and look for opportunities to help others.

When someone is wounded and placed in the hospital or he has surgery, the doctors and nurses get him up and move him nearly immediately after the procedure. Movement and exercise is good for our wounded body parts. I learned the quicker and more my leg was used the better it felt. I kept my range of motion because I stretched and worked my injured leg. Exercising the wound strengthens it. Without movement, we lose range of motion, and we become stiff.

My leg has a scar. It is a distant memory now of what I experienced. The good news is that my leg still works. I can walk, run and jump on it. There are no long-term effects. I am a bit wiser and a lot more refined than when it happened. I'm in a much better position now to help others or warn them of potentially hurtful situations. My life has moved forward and so will yours. Believe it or not, your wound will not be a long-term, debilitating injury. You will make it through this! Just as a bad storm comes through and keeps the sunlight out and reeks havok and then gradually leaves, so your miscarriage clouds will eventually dissipate; and you will begin to see the rays of sunlight radiating within your soul.

Copyright © 2009 **MiscarriageSupport.com**

Get Professional Support... call 1-800-275-9105

No matter what I did to heal my leg I could only do so much. There was only so much in my control. I tried to do everything I could to help my leg heal; however, there was no healing possible without a higher power's involvement. You do all that you can, but grace is what does the rest when healing from a miscarriage.

Copyright © 2009 **MiscarriageSupport.com**

Get Professional Support... call 1-800-275-9105

Heavenly Father

We lived with our Heavenly Father as spirit children before we came to this earth. He loved us unconditionally, taught us at His knee and knew us perfectly. Each of us wanted to be like Him, he has a perfected body of flesh and bones and thus we needed to come to earth to obtain a body of flesh and bones and learn to live by faith. It is a place we can be proven and learn lessons of faith and how to become a father and mother ourselves. Our body is required in order to become more like Him; and, thus, a body is one of the main purposes of this life. We receive a body within our mother's womb.

There were many noble and great spirits in our pre-earth life. There were also rebellious spirits just as there are rebellious people here. Some of those spirits who were very special and extremely valiant didn't need to be proven here, as they had developed to such a state in the pre-existence that they had nothing to prove here. However, they did still need to receive a body. I believe Heavenly Father spared them the evils of this world because of their greatness and purity they attained to with Him; and all they needed to do was receive a body, which was accomplished within their mother's womb.

I believe that these amazing spirits were taken back to Heavenly Father. While it is so painful and hard for us to understand their death, He knows all things; and because of His infinite love for us and our little ones, He is protecting them and blessing them because of their obedience.

I trust that each righteous father and mother will have the opportunity to raise these deceased children to adulthood during the millennium. So while this is a very painful-separation from your baby now-know it is only a temporary one if you will strive to be worthy of that blessing in the hereafter.

Copyright © 2009 **MiscarriageSupport.com**

Get Professional Support... call 1-800-275-9105

I would propose that the first and foremost way to begin to heal is to develop and increase your faith in Heavenly Father. I know He loves us and wants to bless us. We don't understand difficult things that happen to us, can bless us with insight and understanding. He does all things for our good and to help us and make us better from the inside out.

Copyright © 2009 MiscarriageSupport.com
Get Professional Support... call 1-800-275-9105

Power Of The Atonement

The power of the atonement is the only power by which I know you can truly heal from a miscarriage. It is the only power to heal from anything. The atonement was carried out by Jesus Christ. He came to earth to bridge the gap for us to be clean so we can return to the presence of our Heavenly Father. There are two parts of His atoning sacrifice that we need to understand to help us through our difficulties.

The first is the Resurrection. Christ broke the bands of death so that all mankind will be resurrected. To be resurrected means to receive our bodies back in perfect form never to die again. Everyone will be resurrected that ever received a body in this life. It is a free gift to everyone, regardless of his character. Both good and bad people in this life will receive their bodies because of Christ's atoning sacrifice and His breaking the bands of death. This includes your miscarried child.

The second is salvation.

Christ also paid for our sins. This is a conditional gift to us based on our repentance. If we are willing to repent of our sins, Christ is willing to take them upon Himself for us because of love. We can be made clean and remove the guilt and pain of sin. If we do not or are not willing to repent of our sins, then we must suffer for them ourselves.

Copyright © 2009 **MiscarriageSupport.com**

Get Professional Support... call 1-800-275-9105

The second part of salvation is Christ's grace or enabling power.

He has not only suffered for sins; but he has also felt all our pains, infirmities, weaknesses, sicknesses, insecurities, abuse and every other possible thing we could go through. He did this in the Garden of Gethsemane so he might know how to succor His people. He could not help us through this life unless He had perfect empathy for what we are going through. He perfectly understands our pain and our broken hearts. He knows exactly what it feels like to experience a miscarriage and to be devastated. Because of this, He also knows how to help us. And help us He will. He is the "Balm of Gilead." He knows how to help heal our hearts and bring peace and understanding to our souls. We must go to Him, learn of Him and try to emulate His perfect character in our lives. To access this enabling power or Grace of the Atonement you simply need:

1. A humble heart. This is very easy after a miscarriage. A broken heart and a contrite spirit are a natural byproduct of a miscarriage.
2. To specifically ask for the enabling power of the Atonement to help you through this tragedy, kneel down and say the words, "Heavenly Father please bless me with the enabling power of the Atonement to help me through this tragedy."

This enabling power or Grace means that on your best day you may be at a three. In order to make it through another day you need to be at an eight. How are you going to make up the five extra places you need? The enabling power of the Atonement will lift you and make you an eight to get through that day. I've experienced this enabling power countless times in my life. The power of the Atonement is what makes us equal to the tasks or challenges before us. We need only to ask Christ to access it. The Atonement can help us be kind to our family when we're angry inside or to be patient with a husband when he doesn't understand. This is a real power that is accessible through asking and living righteously. Christ can make us equal to any task, any crisis and any pain.

As we live worthily, we can have His spirit with us and calm our troubled hearts. The Savior said in the New Testament: "I will not leave you comfortless. … Peace I leave with you, my peace I give unto you: not as the world giveth, give I unto you. Let not your heart be troubled, neither let it be afraid." (John 14:18, 27.)

Copyright © 2009 **MiscarriageSupport.com**

Get Professional Support… call 1-800-275-9105

We knew we could cast our miscarriage burden on the Lord and he would sustain us. I truly believed His promise, "Blessed are they that mourn: for they shall be comforted."(John 22:22) I know this works. If you haven't felt His redeeming influence in your life, I believe it will be so much harder to heal from this tragedy. He brings insight and perspective. To be able to go to someone and express the feelings you have deep in your heart and know He completely understands and He will run to you to help you, brings great comfort. I recommend Him to you and to your family.

Copyright © 2009 **MiscarriageSupport.com**

Get Professional Support... call 1-800-275-9105

Chapter
14

Prayer

There is someone who always understands. Heavenly Father hears and answers prayers. If you will get on your knees and seek Heavenly Father's blessings He will help you. A person is never as tall as when he is on his knees. We have been given our agency; and, thus, Heavenly Father will not force blessings upon us. Just as we have the ability to choose right and wrong, we have the agency to go to Him in prayer and seek His help. When we choose to do so, there is a sweet peace that will come into our lives.

Going through a miscarriage can put a great strain on a marriage. The best way we found to stay close to each other and learn each other's needs was to pray together each morning as husband and wife. To hear your spouse pray for you, for your needs, your worries, your stresses and to tell Heavenly Father how much he loves you will bond you together. For most of my marriage I didn't pray with my wife, we offered our individual prayers separately; but we seldom prayed together. I recommend this as the most powerful healing event of your day!

Copyright © 2009 **MiscarriageSupport.com**

Get Professional Support... call 1-800-275-9105

Potential Reason For Your Miscarriage

Each miscarriage is unique. Each miscarriage is personal and has it's own reason for happening. I don't believe there are any coincidences. There really is a reason for you having a miscarriage. Medically, you may never know details; but spiritually, you can receive revelation helping you to understand the whys. We learned our "why."

A week before our miscarriage, my wife, who is extremely spiritual, came to me and asked for a blessing. A blessing is when a priesthood holder puts his hands upon the head of an individual and through the priesthood of God pronounces a blessing from Heavenly Father to that person. Blessings are very sacred and come directly from Heavenly Father.

In this blessing my wife was told that our unborn child would bless our family for generations. A week later she miscarried. We didn't understand- the Lord had told us this child would be a blessing for generations to our family. How could this be? How could she bless us when she wasn't going to be physically in our home?

Our thoughts went to a scripture: "And now, my dearly beloved brethren and sisters, let me assure you that these are principles in relation to the dead and the living that cannot be lightly passed over, as pertaining to our salvation. For their salvation is necessary and essential to our salvation, as Paul says concerning the fathers—that they without us cannot be made perfect—neither can we without our dead be made perfect."(D&C 128:15)

Copyright © 2009 **MiscarriageSupport.com**

Get Professional Support... call 1-800-275-9105

We understood that while in this life with a mortal body, there are only certain things we can do to have influence upon each other. It is all direct communication- mortal to mortal.

When we die, we have the same interests we now have. We will be just as interested in our families and concerned with their welfare and their righteousness. We need our dead to help us to be made perfect. When we die, our spirits leave our bodies. Those spirits are us; we don't change. That spirit possessing the same interests as on earth has the ability and power to help us in ways it couldn't with a body. That spirit can whisper to our mind and heart. It now communicates spirit to spirit. We can be influenced by thoughts and feelings from relatives who have passed on. Their intentions are to help us, comfort us and bless us.

It was with this understanding we realized that this precious little girl we lost will truly bless our family for generations, but on the other side of the veil. She was *stillborn*-still born on the other side of the veil. She was still born to bless us from the other side. Only now she has no body and can guide and protect us and our posterity through our thoughts and feelings. She can also influence others through thoughts and feelings. She is still alive and serving us daily. We feel her watching over us and know that as hard as it is now to not have her in our home, she is a part of our family and is helping to perfect us in ways in which we constantly need help.

Hope

I hope this book has given you hope! Hope is not a wish. The kind of hope I'm talking about is an assurance of the promises God has given. God has promised you and me He will bless and help us as we strive to keep His commandments. If you are doing that, then the promises are sure. He will not and cannot abandon that. He has promised to send His peace and help you heal from any wound.

Have faith in that.

Even though you currently feel deeply hurt, I want you to know you will feel better. You will be happy again. Your guilt and shame will eventually leave. You

Copyright © 2009 **MiscarriageSupport.com**

Get Professional Support... call 1-800-275-9105

will be yourself again. I want you to know that I know this is true. My family has experienced it and so will yours.

God bless you.

Copyright © 2009 **MiscarriageSupport.com**

Get Professional Support... call 1-800-275-9105

Remember... you have help
Visit our website:

http://www.MiscarriageSupport.com

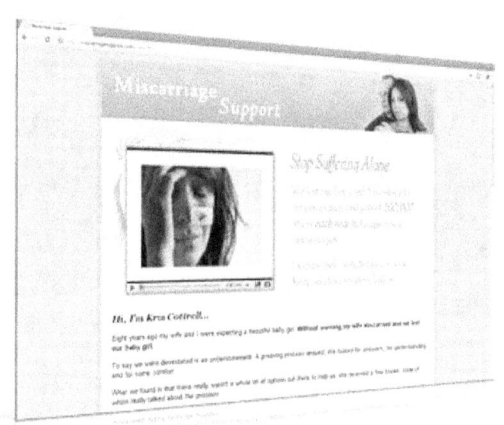 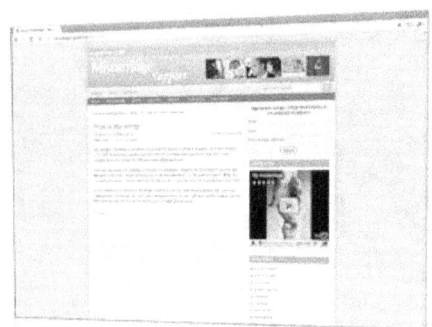

To obtain access to our membership site, please email:

support@miscarriagesupport.com

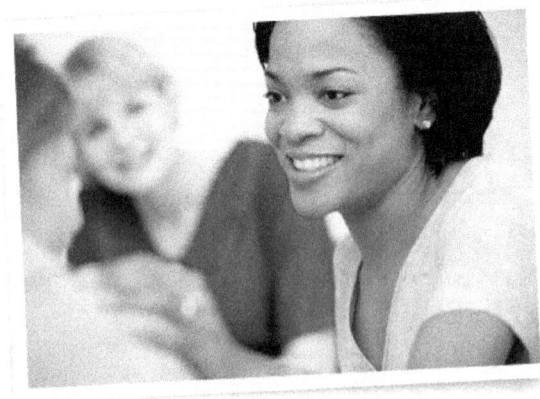

Copyright © 2009 **MiscarriageSupport.com**

Get Professional Support... call 1-800-275-9105

Notes:

Copyright © 2009 MiscarriageSupport.com
Get Professional Support... call 1-800-275-9105

www.ingramcontent.com/pod-product-compliance
Lightning Source LLC
Chambersburg PA
CBHW081127280526
45787CB00007B/3002